Nourish Your Body

JOURNAL TO ELEVATE YOUR LIFE

Using a journal is simply writing down your thoughts and feelings to understand them more clearly. And if you struggle with stress, depression, or anxiety, keeping a journal can help you gain control of your emotions and improve your mental health as well as your your physical health.

ISBN-13: 978-1724832535
ISBN-10: 1724832530

True healing comes
by nourishing the
mind, the body,
and the soul.

Love yourself
enough to live a
healthy lifestyle.

Eat to nourish
your body.

Take care of your body, it's the only place you have to live in.

A healthy lifestyle not only changes your body, it changes your mind, your attitude, and your mood.

Your body can
stand almost
anything, it's your
mind you have to
convince.

The greatest
wealth is health!

Feed the mind
good wisdom, the
body good
nutrition, the soul
good vibes, and the
heart good love.
Elevation for your
situation.
~ T.F. Hodge

The reason one
vitamin can cure
so many diseases is
because a
deficiency in one
vitamin can cause
so many illnesses.
~ Dr. Andrew Saul

You can't enjoy life
if you're not
nourishing your
body.

Remember, when your body is hungry it wants nutrients, not calories.

If you're nourishing your body on the inside, you'll see the results on the outside.

www.ingramcontent.com/pod-product-compliance
Lightning Source LLC
Chambersburg PA
CBHW070132260726
48658CB00001B/369